I0440864

Bye bye IBS! The Natural Irritable Bowel Syndrome Cure

Chapter 1: How do I know if I have Irritable Bowel Syndrome?..page 3

Chapter 2: What Causes Irritable Bowel Syndrome?..page 5

Chapter 3: How to Heal Your Colon……………..…..page 7

Chapter 4: Foods to Avoid…………..……………....page 14

Chapter 5: How to Feel Great, Stay Healthy, and Have Energy……………………………………………...page 28

Chapter 6: Maintaining Your Cure………………..…page 35

Hello and welcome. If you are experiencing Irritable Bowel Syndrome (IBS) I have felt like you feel now. I know what gave me permanent relief, and I'm here to share what I have learned. So take a nice, long, slow breath through your nose and slowly breathe it out knowing that soon you will be able to stop your IBS as I did.

With Love,
 Joel Blanchard

How do I know if I have Irritable Bowel Syndrome?

Irritable Bowel Syndrome is also known as "mucous colitis," "spastic colon," and "irritable colon." Whatever you call it, this condition is so common that it affects about twenty-three percent of adults. This condition is characterized by chronic gut discomfort, ranging from quite mild to very acute. Some of the symptoms of IBS include abdominal cramping, abdominal pain, excessive gas, nausea, headache, constipation, diarrhea, blood or mucus in stools and a feeling of fullness in the belly. Although these symptoms, in and of themselves, are not life-threatening, having IBS symptoms often means that you have an unhealthy colon, and THAT absolutely DOES pose several threats to your long-term health. Colon problems can lead to eczema, heart disease, chronic fatigue, diabetes, arthritis, autism, ulcerative colitis and even cancer. If you have a problem with your colon you have an immune system problem. It is consistently estimated that 70-80% of your immune system is located in your digestive system. The vast majority of your serotonin is manufactured in your intestines as well, so it's not at all surprising that if you have an unhealthy gut you won't be happy about it!

Most Western Medicine practitioners (the majority of U.S. doctors) will tell you that there is no specific blood test, X-ray or scan that can conclusively determine that you are suffering from IBS. Their diagnosis is usually made by evaluating your symptoms. They may be able to offer other blood tests, or more intrusive tests to rule out other conditions, but from what I've heard from my clients, they usually don't use the proper tools to examine your colon in the proper way. Most doctors will tell you that irritable bowel syndrome is not curable.

I am required to say that if you are suffering from a medical condition you should visit or consult with your health care provider. Fortunately, I still have the freedom to say that I believe that you know yourself better than anyone else. I have the utmost faith in you to be able to tell whether you are feeling well or not, narrow down the probable cause(s) of your illness, and decide what path to the cure you wish to take.

So if you're wondering if you have Irritable Bowel Syndrome, let me ask you these questions:

Have your bowel habits changed?

Do you experience abdominal pain and/or bloating?

Do you feel as though you have excessive gas and/or your flatulence is unusually smelly?

Do you have nausea before or after bowel movements?

Is your pain temporarily relieved after having bowel movements?

Do you often experience pain soon after eating?

Are you passing blood or mucus in your bowel movements? (Note: blood in stools may be caused by many conditions. If this is your primary symptom you really should have tests taken to exclude other conditions)

Are you often constipated and have to strain to have a bowel movement?

Do you often have diarrhea?

Do you have headaches or does your mind feel cloudy like you can't think straight?

Do you suffer from depression and/or anxiety? (If you are suffering from panic or anxiety attacks you should acquire a copy of my e-book entitled "The Complete Anxiety and Panic Attack Cure.")

If you answered "Yes" to several of these questions you are probably suffering from the condition called Irritable Bowel Syndrome. So now, what you should want to know is what is causing you to have this condition.

What Causes Irritable Bowel Syndrome?

Your large and small intestines, together, measure about 26 feet long, and they twist and turn all over your abdomen. Your small intestine is relatively narrow, is about 21 feet long, and is located below your ribcage and above your waistline. There are many tiny, finger-like structures on the inside of your small intestine called microvilli (or "villi" for short). These villi, along with folds in the intestine wall, help you absorb nutrients from the food you eat. Unfortunately all these twists and turns and folds in a long narrow tube are subject to blockages, bulging pockets of excrement, and narrowed, spastic constrictions.

Your large intestine is about five feet long and is wider in diameter than your small intestine. Your large intestine rises up on the right side of your abdomen, lies across your body and descends on the left side of your abdomen. Your large intestine is full of bacteria. Some of these bacteria help to break down proteins. Your large intestine is also used to store feces before it is defecated out of your body. Unfortunately the kinds and amounts of bacteria in the large intestine can get out of balance, and usually do, especially if you've ever been on antibiotics.

So what you simply need to realize is that your colon, like most things, needs some kind of maintenance. What would your skin look like if you never washed it? What would your sink and toilet look like if you never cleaned them? If you haven't cleaned your colon for years and years you have likely accumulated impacted waste in your colon. This impacted fecal material becomes hard and compacted, and sticks to the walls of your colon, effectively inhibiting your villi from doing its job. When your microvilli stop working properly you are unable to properly extract the vitamins, minerals, and other nutrients from your food, and those nutrients are not available for your body. Blocked or damaged villi are not able to do their job of helping to keep waste material moving along smoothly in your intestines.

If you were eating a perfectly organic, whole-food diet, like a wild animal, your colon might stay healthy. Unfortunately, if you have been eating the Standard American Diet (S.A.D.), or even something close to it, you are introducing all kinds of toxins into your colon. Even if you're eating fairly well, it is estimated that there are over 300,000 different toxins that have been found in the air and water of the Earth. These toxins can injure the colon and stick to the colon walls, encouraging more blockages and making the colon narrower. Some side effects of an impa red colon are bloating, cramping and excess gas. A significantly narrowed or blocked colon can lead to acne, constipation, irritable bowel syndrome, and ultimately, disease.

In addition to seriously weakening your immune system, an impaired colon is also directly linked to anxiety, stress and depression because about 95% of your serotonin is produced in your gut. Serotonin is sometimes referred to as the "happy hormone" because it helps to evoke your sense of well-being in the brain. An imbalance in serotonin can cause depression, anxiety, sleep problems, mood swings, and changes in your appetite for food or sex. IBS literally makes people sad.

Would you like to know how you can heal your colon and stop experiencing any problem caused by an unhealthy colon? I hope so!

How to Heal Your Colon

Your colon requires three main things in order to work properly: a healthy diet, periodic cleanses, and periodic infusions of good bacteria (probiotics). Ideally you will commit to all three of these elements. Giving your body good bacteria could be as simple as taking a probiotic pill, but even a high quality probiotic pill will do little good if your colon is clogged up and you continue to eat bad bacteria and toxins. I will talk in great detail about what to eat and what not to eat later in this book. For now just think of a healthy diet as one consisting of whole, non-processed foods like organic fruit and vegetables, and raw nuts and seeds. Microwaved corn dogs are not on the list, sorry.

To start getting immediate relief from your irritable bowel syndrome, however, I recommend that you get your hands on some slippery elm bark (ulmus fulva). Whenever I got cramps or nausea I would take two capsules of slippery elm bark and my symptoms would subside within 15 minutes. Slippery elm is an extremely safe herb, and it has a mucilaginous effect on the linings of the stomach and intestines (that's a good thing). Slippery elm coats and protects mucous membranes such as those found in the gastrointestinal tract. Slippery elm bark has been shown to effectively soothe inflamed or irritated stomach and intestinal wall linings. Frontier Natural Products markets an excellent organic slippery elm inner bark powder, and there are several reputable companies that offer capsules of slippery elm bark; these companies include Solaray, Nature's Way, Nature's Herbs and Nature's Answer. Head to the closest health food store and get some, or order some online, and do it soon! Slippery elm bark is most effective between meals or at least twenty minutes after eating.

Another supplement to pick up to start healing your gut is some L-glutamine powder. L-glutamine has been proven to help repair damaged intestines. In fact, L-glutamine is perhaps the most important nutrient for the integrity of your intestinal walls and serves as an energy source for your immune system. I suggest using a pure L-glutamine powder, but capsules are also okay. Take 2,000mg (2 grams) two or three times a day on a truly empty stomach. Before you go to sleep is a good time to take L-glutamine if you don't eat immediately before sleeping. It's a good idea to not eat right before sleeping anyway, because it gives your digestive tract more time to rest and heal each night.

If you're suffering from heartburn or gastro esophageal reflux disease (GERD), drink one ounce of organic Aloe Vera juice (made from inner filet) in-between meals and take a digestive enzyme supplement right before meals. Aloe Vera can sooth the symptoms of irritated bowels and helps to keep your digestive system healthy. It neutralizes stomach acid naturally, so it's a wonderful remedy to use instead of commercial antacids that often contain ingredients that I wouldn't want in my body. Good digestive enzyme supplements, like Natural Factor's "Dr. Murray's Multi Enzyme", contain the enzymes protease to digest protein, amylase to digest carbohydrates, and lipase to digest fats. These enzymes can make it a lot easier for your body to break food down and they help give your pancreas a rest. By breaking down food into smaller pieces it is easier for your intestines to handle the food, and makes it easier for your body to deliver nutrients from the food into your bloodstream. Your pancreas can only make a limited amount of enzymes, and if you have been eating anything other than raw food (and who hasn't right!?) your pancreas has been working hard to produce enzymes to digest those foods. Heartburn is a common symptom of enzyme deficiency because without the enzymatic catalyst for the digestive reaction to take place, virtually all your body can do is throw more hydrochloric acid (HCL or stomach acid) at the food in your stomach.

If you're constipated you should increase your magnesium intake because magnesium draws water to your bowels. The U.S. Recommended Daily Allowance (RDA) for magnesium is 6 mg per kilogram of body weight, which translates to 420 mg for a 70 Kg person. A kilogram is about 2.2 pounds. Most people are severely magnesium deficient. Many people can feel their muscles and body relax when they take magnesium, so you might want to wait until you're home for the evening before you take it. If I were constipated I would take 400 milligrams (mg) of magnesium citrate or magnesium aspartate immediately and then take 200 milligrams every hour or two later until my bowels moved. Even if you're not constipated it's a good idea to take about 2 milligrams for every pound you weigh before you go to bed. If you weigh 150 pounds take about 300 milligrams of magnesium every night.

Beware! Most of the colon products that you find in drugstores, supermarkets and even health food stores are arguably bad for you. Most of these products are merely laxatives or suppositories, and laxatives and suppositories do not cleanse impacted fecal matter well at all. There are all types of laxatives, ranging from ones that draw water to your intestines, stimulate your intestines or add bulk (usually in the form of fiber) into your intestines.

Laxatives can cause the following negative results...
Dehydration
Addiction (a.k.a. Lazy Bowel Syndrome)
Electrolyte imbalances
Allergic reactions
Cramping
Decreased nutrient absorption
Bloating
Diarrhea
Blockages in the intestines
Loss of intestinal muscle strength

Even "natural" laxatives like guar gum, senna, and psyllium are not recommended. Guar gum can cause nausea and intestinal blockages, senna may be toxic to your liver and/or damage the lining of your colon, and psyllium can cause severe allergic reactions and intestinal blockages. When I worked as a Public Nutritionist I would often hear people with compromised intestinal linings complain that psyllium caused them significant abdominal discomfort.

Let's pretend that you've already gone to the grocery store and filled your shelves with organic, healthy food (which you are now eating), and you are ready to do a cleanse. There are many ways to clean your colon, but some are decidedly better than others.

A proper colon cleanse can...
Remove impacted fecal matter from pockets in your colon and reduce bloating
Remove fecal matter from the walls of your intestines and allow better nutrition intake
Decrease the time it takes for food to pass through your intestines, reducing rancidity and toxins
Enable more frequent elimination
Enable more thorough elimination
Prevent constipation
Stop Irritable Bowel Syndrome symptoms
Help normalize your nerves in your intestines and appendix
Reduce candida yeast overgrowth

Reduce the buildup of bad bacteria
Reduce or eliminate intestinal parasites
Provide a nurturing environment for good bacteria (probiotics)
Help reduce stress and depression by promoting serotonin production in the colon
Decrease the irritation of your colon lining
Alleviate gas, bloating, cramping, and pain
Decrease your body weight by about 5-20 pounds, because that's how much fecal matter most Americans have stuck in their large intestines

You want to experience those benefits right? Let me tell you how I actually stopped experiencing the symptoms of irritable bowel syndrome forever. First I improved my diet, then I got my colon cleaned out using hydrotherapy (also known as a high colonic or colon irrigation), and then I restored my probiotic (good bacteria) balance. I know that most people dread the thought of having anything inserted in their rectum, or talking about these sorts of things with others, but please understand that the people who administer hydrotherapy are often professionals who formerly suffered from intestinal problems themselves. You don't need to have insurance to have a high colonic cleaning done and sessions usually cost between fifty and eighty dollars. Hydrotherapy (colonic irrigation) is a process of using clean water to clean out your colon. Warm, purified water is introduced into your colon via your rectum. It fills your colon slowly and then slowly flows back out a tube. The water makes your colon produce a muscular contraction called peristalsis, which can help your body get rid of fecal matter, gas, bacteria, undigested food, mucous, and parasites that have built up in the colon. This procedure can clean out fecal matter that has been stuck in your colon for years. You should never experience any pain or great discomfort during this procedure, and no drugs are required. Multiple hydrotherapy sessions may be required to thoroughly clean out your colon. Please search your phone book or look on the internet for a high colonic clinic in your area. The therapist there should be licensed, patient, and answer any questions you might have. If you don't feel comfortable with that particular therapist then contact another office, but don't rule out this shortcut to quick, effective colon cleansing.

Colon therapy (Hydrotherapy) is not recommended for people with:
    congestive heart failure
    diverticulitis (current infection)

ulcerative colitis
crohn's disease
severe or internal hemorrhoids
tumors in the rectum or colon
intestinal perforation
carcinoma of the rectum
fissures or fistula
severe hemorrhoids
painful abdominal hernia
renal insufficiency
recent colon or rectal surgery
cirrhosis of the liver
or are in the first or last trimester of pregnancy

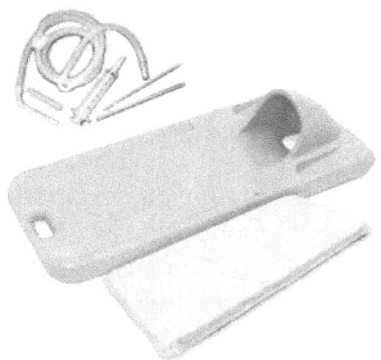

A colema board

If you cannot find a high colonic specialist in your area, or choose not to employ one, you can actually do a similar procedure at home using what's called a colema board. To use a colema board you need to position yourself over a toilet using the board and a chair. You can purchase colema boards online for about $280 and they usually come with the necessary tubing, disposable rectal tips and instructions. You will also need a large bucket to hold the clean irrigating water.

Hydrotherapy cleans much more deeply than a regular enema can. Enemas usually consist of water or a saline solution being introduced into the rectum. These types of enemas only help to remove waste in the lowest part of the colon. Enemas can be made to be more effective by introducing herbs, bentonite clay, oils, oxygen-based colon cleansers or organic coffee into the fluid injected, but they do not cleanse enough of the intestinal tract to serve our purpose here. Speak with your hydrotherapy practitioner if you wish any of those additives to be added to the water used to flush you out during your high colonic sessions.

If you do not wish to undergo hydrotherapy I suggest that you at least do a colon cleanse using a product like Nature's Secret Ultimate Cleanse. This is a well-designed product which can remove waste and toxins from your colon. I have used this product and it worked well for me. This product has cascara sagrada in it. The anthraquinone glycosides in cascara sagrada help to purge your bowels of waste by increasing peristalsis (muscular contraction) in the lower bowel. Cascara sagrada can, however, be quite addictive, so be sure to only use this product for no more than 30 days and then discontinue use.

Remember, eating a diet composed of primarily whole, organic fruit and vegetables is the best way to keep your digestive tract clean and healthy from the top down. This diet should be employed before, during and after any colon cleaning.

After your colon has been cleansed it's very important to take a good, full-spectrum probiotic (good bacteria) product. Many IBS patients have been found to have helicobacter pylori, blastocystis hominis, or dientamoeba fragilis bacteria overgrowth; probiotics fight against those bad bacteria. Probiotics also help you digest your food, produce and absorb vitamins and minerals, and help your body get rid of toxins. Don't make the mistake of thinking that your body has enough good bacteria because you eat yogurt. The kind of yogurt most people consume, commercial yogurt, is not recommended at all. A single serving of commercial yogurt usually has only about 500,000 good bacteria cells in it. A good probiotic pill will have about fifteen million good bacteria organisms living in it, thirty times as much as the yogurt. Also, commercial yogurts are often fermented for only a few hours, can contain detrimental hormones such as rHBT, and are sometimes loaded with sugar. I strongly suggest that you take a full-spectrum probiotic, meaning that it contains several different bacteria strains, not just acidophilus and bifidus. Some good probiotics are Natural Factor's Ultimate Probiotic 12-12, Udo's Choice Super 8 Probiotic, and Dr. Mercola's Complete Probiotics.

After cleaning your colon you can help keep it clean by periodically eating some bentonite clay. Bentonite clay has been eaten for thousands of years, and can help remove chemical, bacterial, and heavy metal toxins from your intestines. This clay is negatively charged, so it attracts, and binds to, the positively charged toxins, helping you to pass them right out of your body.

Foods to Avoid

There are many foods that encourage irritable bowel syndrome symptoms. The most common substances that exacerbate IBS are sugar, lactose, gluten and the wrong kinds of fats. Allergens in food are another common cause of ongoing colon and body inflammation. Almost all food allergies are caused by just eight kinds of food: dairy, eggs, peanuts, tree nuts, soy, wheat, fish and shellfish. Dairy products often cause cramping and worsen IBS symptoms. If you pay close attention to how you feel after eating pasteurized milk or cheese you will almost certainly feel the negative effects of these foods. The pasteurization and homogenization process essentially ruins the benefits milk, denaturing any proteins or minerals present, and killing all of the live enzymes and probiotics that the milk originally contained. While it's relatively easy to avoid things like nuts and shellfish, wheat is especially difficult to avoid because it is in so many processed foods. The gliadin content of wheat gluten can cause the production of Immunoglobulin A, Immunoglobulin G and Immunoglobulin M, the antibodies that your body produces in response to what it considers to be foreign or dangerous body invaders. These antibodies, like histamine, irritate and inflame your body. Wheat and rye are responsible for a great deal of body inflammation, and sensitivities to the allergens in these foods can cause irritable bowel syndrome. A protein in coffee can "cross-react" with gluten so you may wish to avoid both regular and decaffeinated coffee if you are quite sensitive to gluten.

I think that nowadays most people are aware that most processed foods are not healthy for their bodies. The VAST majority of the foods sold at a typical American grocery store actually encourage irritable bowel syndrome symptoms. Once you know the facts about the ways these foods are processed, and the chemicals in them, I think that you will want to start avoiding these foods for several reasons.

Not eating foods that are detrimental to your body is as important as eating foods that are good for your body. I'm about to talk about a lot of different foods that I know are not good for you. There are often several reasons why each one of the foods that I'm about to discuss is not good for you; I'm not going to mention every reason, as that would probably not hold your attention anyway. My goal here is to simply point out foods to avoid and give you at least one, solid reason as to why you should avoid them. Currently much of the research done on these "bad" foods is sponsored by the companies that manufacture them, and the studies are carefully crafted to produce results that make the foods appear safe or benign. If the results of any of their sponsored studies don't turn out the way these companies want they simply do not report those results to any media and you will never hear about those studies. Other times, completely accurate results of studies are delivered to the media, results that would alert millions of people to the hazards of popular foods, and the media either does not air that story or puts a "spin" on the findings to dilute its impact. My point is that I REGULARLY hear or read information about food, supplements and nutrition from media sources that are outright lies. Fortunately there have been some unbiased laboratory studies done, and these studies clearly demonstrate how dangerous some popular foods are and how healing some foods are. I sought out and scrutinized these research studies during the years that I worked as a Nutritional Advisor, and I still seek out these studies today. I have also used my personal experience of working with thousands of people suffering and recovering from virtually every type of body affliction known to humankind to see first-hand which foods truly heal and which foods truly cause harm.

The Threat: Hydrogenated oils

The hydrogenation process changes the fatty acids in foods into malformed, chemically modified fatty acids. From a nutritional standpoint the hydrogenation process turns usable essential fats into unusable fats that confuse and harm your body. For example, your body uses fatty acids to form the walls of every cell in your body. When those cell walls are made out of the wrong form of fat they are liable to not function properly; they may fail to keep bad things out of the cell and fail to allow good things in, and are much more likely to rupture, causing cell death.

A study performed in 2001 showed that hydrogenated oil had an adverse effect on cardiovascular disease and contributed to atherogenesis (the formation of abnormal fatty or lipid masses on arterial walls) (Sung Ham, et. al, 2001). Even partial hydrogenation turns unsaturated fatty acids into highly toxic trans fatty acids (trans-isomer fatty acids) and other "altered fat substances," many of which haven't even been studied yet. Diets high in trans fatty acids tend to cause weight gain and diabetes as it is difficult for your body to get rid of this junk and your body will still "feel like" eating fat because it still doesn't have the quality essential fats it needs. IBS sufferers especially should avoid eating a diet high in in this kind of fat.

Food manufacturers are required to list on the label if a food contains more than 0.5 grams of trans fat per serving, so be sure to read labels. Just be aware that the manufacturers often make the serving size so small that the food is now under 0.5 grams "per serving" and the trans fat is not listed.

Here is a list of some of the foods that contain high levels of hydrogenated oil.

Avoid this stuff!

Margarine - Most margarine is virtually pure hydrogenated oil. It's better to use organic butter (forget about the lies you've heard about butter being so bad for you - we'll talk about the healthy fats found in butter later) or a quality vegan spread.

Doughnuts, Hamburger Buns, Hotdog buns, most Tortillas and most Breads - Most breads, buns, tortillas and other things made out of flour contain high amounts of hydrogenated oil and undergo a horrific processing procedure. Most commercial flour is bleached with a toxic bleaching agent, such as chlorine, which destroys many of the vitamins that were originally present in the flour. Buying whole grain breads that do not contain "enriched" flour is better, but I'm going to point out the problems with wheat later, so don't stock up on whole wheat either. Doughnuts are one of the worst things you could possibly eat; they contain hydrogenated oils, white flour, sugar, and acrylamides. Acrylamides are carcinogenic constituents that get created when foods are grilled, fried, baked or roasted.

Vegetable Shortening - Vegetable shortening is full of hydrogenated oils. In some recipes you can use palm oil or coconut oil instead of shortening, especially for temperatures not exceeding 300 degrees.

French Fries, Fried Chicken, and most other Fried Foods - You probably figured I'd get around to telling you not to eat "fast food" sooner or later right?! Fried foods are often loaded with unhealthy, carcinogenic (cancer-causing) fat and lots of low-nutrient calories. Fried foods usually contain acrylamides. Foods such as French fries, potato chips, toasted breads and grilled meats and vegetables often contain these cancer-causing byproducts.

Non-Dairy Whipped Dessert Toppings, Non-Dairy Creamers, Cake Frosting and

Cake Mixes - These foods are often very high in trans fats. You can use quality vegan toppings, vegan coffee creamers or coconut milk powder. Make a healthy organic fruit pie instead of a cake; the cake mix itself is usually toxic.

Commercial Peanut Butter - The vast majority of peanut butter sold in stores have unacceptably high amounts of hydrogenated oil. Other than grinding peanuts yourself, there are prepackaged peanut butters that are made out only 100% organic peanuts [and salt if you want]... isn't that what you want?

Commercial Vegetable Oils - Many vegetable oils (vegetable oils are plant triglycerides that are liquid at room temperature) are chemically treated, oxidized and are partially hydrogenated. About 97% of the fat in the human body is saturated and monounsaturated fat and only about 3 % is polyunsaturated fats. Vegetable oils often contain high levels of polyunsaturated fats, especially omega-6, which isn't what your body needs a lot of. Omega-3 fatty acids are beneficial polyunsaturated fats that our bodies need but are usually deficient in, and the polyunsaturated fat in vegetable oils crowds out omega-3 and ruins our omega-3 to omega-6 ratio (which should be close to 1:1). Excessive omega-6 fat has been linked to cancer (Hughes-Fulford, M., et al., 2006). Additionally, the polyunsaturated fats found in vegetable oils are highly unstable and oxidize easily. These types of oxidized fats can cause inflammation (that can clog arteries), cell mutation (which plays a large factor in cancer) and deplete your body of beneficial antioxidants.

Commercial Salad dressings, Mayonnaise and other Condiments - Not only are these foods full of calories and low in nutrients, but they often contain hydrogenated, genetically modified corn or soybean oil. "Light" or "low-fat" mayonnaise is even unhealthier than regular mayonnaise because, in addition to the soybean oil found in most mayonnaise, these versions often contain genetically modified corn starch, phosphoric acid and preservatives such as sodium benzoate. A fresh salad dressing is easy to make at home using quality olive oil and apple cider vinegar (along with your favorite seasonings), and can actually help your body absorb more of the nutrients present in the salad greens.

Crackers, Cereals, Cookies, Chips and "Snack Foods"- Most commercial crackers, cereals cookies, chips and "snacks" contain partially hydrogenated soybean oil or partially hydrogenated cottonseed oil. Avoid anything made with cottonseed oil. Cottonseed oil is high in saturated fat and often contains high levels of pesticides and natura ly occurring toxins.

Ice Cream - Most ice cream contains hydrogenated vegetable, soybean, palm, and/or other types of oil. Check the labels because some ice cream does not contain these ingredients. Ice cream is not good for you. Ice cream usually contains fat, sugar, cholesterol, casein, lactose, no fiber and extremely few nutrients relative to its calorie content.

Frozen dinners - Most frozen dinners contain some type of hydrogenated oil, genetically modified ingredients, and are often high in the wrong kind of fats as well.

The Threat: Foods derived from Genetically Modified Organisms

According to the Grocery Manufacturers of America, in 2009, approximately 70 percent of the foods on grocery store shelves were manufactured using genetically modified organisms (GMOs). From my direct observation, the percentage of products in the average U.S. grocery store containing genetically modified organisms is now over 80%! I don't know of any large fast food restaurant chain that does not have genetically altered crops in its food. Every person in the United States, who is not consistently seeking out products that do not contain GMOs, is eating GMOs.

Genetically modified organisms are laboratory-produced organisms that have had changes made to their DNA (genes have been inserted into, or deleted from, their natural deoxyribonucleic acid chain). I first heard about GMO's in the 90's when Monsanto released GM plants that were resistant to their herbicide (plant-killer) RoundUp. The idea was that a farmer could plant a field of these GM herbicide-resistant plants and then spray the entire field with RoundUp to kill any weeds or competing plants. The plan worked fairly well, but now you had a field of crops that had been sprayed with an herbicide containing glyphosate. When you spray glyphosate on a plant it becomes systemic throughout the plant, it cannot be washed off, and if you eat this plant the glyphosate ends up in your body. Glyphosate in your intestines can kill your beneficial bacteria (probiotics) which is a serious threat to your health. One of the most important things that I've come to realize over the years is that the ratio of good to bad bacteria in your gut has a huge impact on your overall health. Also, glyphosate can significantly reduce the amount of beneficial micronutrients, such as manganese and zinc, in plants because it acts as a chelator. In the United States, approximately 86% of the corn is genetically modified, about 91% of the soybeans are genetically modified and about 93% of the cotton is genetically modified.

Most genetically modified corn and cotton are designed so that they produce their own pesticide known as the Bt-toxin (the CryAb1 toxin from Bacillus thuringiensis). The Bt-toxin is inside the plant itself and cannot be washed off. When pests eat the corn or cotton containing this insecticidal protein the poison splits their stomachs open and kills them. This poison is not good for your stomach or intestines either!

The really scary thing is that even if you stop eating these GM foods the harmful proteins they contain may continue to be produced inside your body because there is evidence that the genes inserted into the GMO may transfer to the bacteria living inside you. Most people assume that genetically modified organisms must be safe because people are already eating them, but the truth is that no trustworthy scientific study has ever shown genetically modified food to be completely safe. In fact, several countries, including Japan, Peru, New Zealand and Switzerland, have completely outlawed GMOs. In 2011, a comprehensive review was made which examined 19 studies in which mammals were fed genetically modified soybeans and corn. This review, conducted by Gilles-Eric Séralini, Robin Mesnage et al. (2011), concluded that a diet of GM food can lead to liver and kidney problems. To learn more about the potential negative health risks of genetically modified food please visit http://www.responsibletechnology.org/gmo-dangers/65-health-risks.

How to Avoid GMO Foods:
Since the vast majority of food sold at the typical American grocery store contains GMOs you must be very careful what you purchase there. **High fructose corn syrup (HFCS) is almost always derived from GM corn, so avoid any food with that ingredient in it**. Avoid any corn or soy product that is not certified organic. By definition, organic products can NOT contain genetically modified ingredients; this is one of the reasons why people are willing to pay more money for organic products. Other major sources of genetically modified organisms and pesticides include cottonseed and canola oil. Also beware of certain varieties of (non-organic) crookneck squash, zucchini and papayas. Most soy (including soy lecithin) is genetically modified and aspartame (NutraSweet) is derived from GMOs.

An easy way to avoid GMOs (and to eat healthy) is to routinely avoid processed, pre-packaged foods and stock up on foods in the produce section. Although I try to grow as much of my own food as I can, when I used to work in a "health food" store I saw that much of the fruits and vegetables being sold were from local farmers and of good quality. At the supermarket, pay close attention to the stickers on the produce. Organic produce has a five digit product code that starts with 9 ("nine" is fine). Genetically modified produce have a five digit product code that starts with 8 ("eight" we hate), but in places with no GMO labeling laws these stickers are often not on the produce. Conventional produce (produce that may have been grown using chemical fertilizers and pesticides but is not GM) has a four digit product code starting with a 4. If you're at a supermarket and there is no sticker on the produce you can be quite certain that it is not organic unless specifically labeled as such (in the United States you can look for the green and white "USDA Organic" label). The problem with conventional produce is that it hasn't necessarily been grown under ideal conditions, may be lower in nutrients than organically produced produce (perhaps limited to the nitrogen-phosphorus-potassium [N-P-K] and random array of trace minerals contained in chemical fertilizers), and may contain significant amounts of hazardous pesticides. One of the easiest ways to always have some kind of healthy food at home is to buy some frozen organic fruits and vegetables and only eat them when you run out of fresh produce. The easiest way to eat healthy is to buy healthy food because, for the most part, you eat what you buy.

The Threat: Excessive Sugar & High Fructose Corn Syrup

The most common substance that exacerbates IBS is probably sugar, in all of its forms. Excessive consumption of simple sugars, like corn syrup, can reduce the positive effects of polysaccharides. On average, people are eating way too much processed sugar. Most 12 ounce sodas, or other sweetened beverages, contain about 40 grams of sugar - that's WAY too much! According to the U.S. Department of Agriculture (USDA) the average American eats about 156 pounds of added sugar each year. As a nutritionist, I'm not the least bit surprised to hear that the incidence of diabetes type 2 continues to rise. Excessive simple sugar consumption leads to insulin resistance, and insulin resistance is the cause of diabetes and several other chronic "diseases." Scientific studies have suggested that excessive fructose consumption encourages over 70 different diseases and/or health problems. When you eat fruit you put a fairly large amount of fructose in your body, but the negative effects to your body due to fructose are mitigated by the fact that you're also getting fiber, vitamins, minerals and other phytonutrients [phytonutrients are all of the other things in foods - many of which researchers haven't even studied yet. Scientists haven't really come close to figuring out the genius of nature yet.]. It's **refined** sugar that you should seek to eliminate from your diet. Even fruit juice should generally be avoided as it is a "refined" product that now contains fructose in a form that your body can absorb very quickly. Many commercial juices have pesticide residue and nasty fungicides and preservatives in them. Almost all commercial juices are pasteurized, further destroying any life-promoting property the juice may have previously contained. Set a goal that you will keep your **refined** sugar intake below 25 grams per day. Beyond all the negative effects sugar has on your body, be aware that high fructose corn syrup is bad for you for other reasons. High fructose corn syrup (aka HFCS, glucose-fructose syrup, glucose/fructose, and high fructose maize syrup) is laboratory-created syrup. Through the use of enzymes some of the glucose in the original corn syrup is converted into fructose. Most of the sweetened foods in America, such as soda, use HFCS 55 which is about 55% fructose and about 42% glucose. In the 1970's food and beverage manufacturers in the United States began switching their default sweetener from sucrose (table sugar) to corn syrup because it saved them a lot of money; high fructose corn syrup is sweeter and less expensive than table sugar. Unfortunately, corn syrup is almost always made out of genetically modified corn, so it contains all the toxins inherent in GM corn (Bt toxin, pesticide and herbicides residues, etc.). Even "regular" processed sugar often contains pesticides. Brazil recently acquired the dubious title of being the world's largest consumer of pesticides, spending an estimated 7 billion dollars on pesticides in one year, primarily for its two largest cash crops – genetically modified soybeans and sugarcane. Most people would lose a significant amount of excessive bodyweight, improve the health of their colons, and feel better simply by reducing their sugar intake.

How to Avoid Refined Sugars
Many processed foods such as cereals, yogurts, snack bars and powdered mixes contain a lot of refined sugar. Even whole foods like dates, figs and prunes may contain too much fructose to be eaten on a regular basis. In short, you need to read labels, avoid sweetened products, not add sugar to things and try to lose your "sweet tooth." If you are able to lose your craving and desire for sweet foods you won't think about them or miss them. I admit that this is not easy to do. Even if you don't think of yourself as someone who eats a lot of sweets I bet that you'd crave sugar if you ate ONLY low-glycemic vegetables, meat and water for 4 months. I know because I did that. In 1995, after western medicine was

unable to solve my intestinal and allergy problems, I visited a Doctor of Chinese Medicine. He quickly diagnosed me as having a massive candida yeast overgrowth in my colon, which was causing my gut and allergy problems. He told me to take probiotics (good bacteria), reduce fatty foods from my diet and cut all the sugar out of my diet for 90 days in order to reduce the number of yeast cells inside me (candida yeast feeds on sugar, thrives in a sluggish colon and competes against good bacteria). I researched candida yeast and decided that I would follow his advice. For four months I literally ate only low-sugar vegetables (such as broccoli, cauliflower, asparagus, lettuce and spinach) and lean meat. No condiments, no fruit, no dairy, no starchy or high-glycemic vegetables (potatoes, parsnips, beet, carrots, peas…etc.) - nothing else except water and maybe some salt or pepper. I was amazed at how much I craved something sweet! But my willpower was strong, and every time I craved sugar I just thought about how the candida yeast inside me wanted sugar, and I was able to harden my resolve and stay on my diet. I continued to crave sugar for about three months but after that I didn't really mind the diet and stayed on it for another month just to make sure that most of the candida yeast in my colon had died off. The diet totally worked, by the way. Not only did it cure my cramping, allergies and candida yeast problems, it changed my life more than anything had ever changed my life before. Once the toxic by-products of candida yeast (which includes acetaldehyde) stopped corrupting my body and blood I was able to think clearly again for the first time since I was a young teenager. I am not however, recommending that you follow this diet; this was done for a specific, therapeutic purpose and is not a diet that would be healthy to stay on long-term. If the average American was forced to eat a truly low sugar diet (i.e. less than 8 grams of sugar a day) they would probably experience such strong detoxification symptoms that they would not be able to handle it. When you stop overwhelming your body with useless calories and low-nutrient food your body has the energy to start healing and detoxifying itself. This is a good thing, but detoxification is something that needs to be done gradually. So for now, just say "no" to sweetened beverages and obviously sugar-laden foods. Eating whole fruits is okay.

The Threat: Artificial sweeteners

You may think that an easy way to avoid fructose, sucrose and glucose is to use products with artificial sweeteners in them such as diet soda…etc. I strongly advise against this. In my opinion, the information that soda manufacturers and artificial sweetener manufacturers spend billions of dollars to propagate through their various websites and advertisements is misleading to say the least. The health risks of artificial sweeteners range from unknown to severe. Let's examine some of the most popular "sugar substitutes" in more detail...

Aspartame (aka Equal, NutraSweet, Spoonful, Amino Sweet)

Aspartame is composed of 10% Methanol, 40% Aspartic Acid and 50% Phenylalanine. Methanol, also known as wood alcohol, is a toxin. As little as 30 milliliters of pure methanol is lethal. Your body absorbs methanol very well and, because it is difficult to excrete, it is regarded as a cumulative toxin. When you ingest methanol it is metabolized in the liver to form formaldehyde and subsequently, formic acid. Methanol may cause pancreatitis, neuropathy, blindness and liver damage (Hantson, P., et al, 2002) (Kapur, B. M., et al, 2007). Aspartame may actually CAUSE diabetes mellitus (type 2) and exacerbates certain side effects of diabetes such as cataracts, diabetic neuropathy, and diabetic retinopathy. A study in 2006 concluded that aspartame was a multi-potential carcinogenic [cancer-causing] agent (Belpoggi, F., et al). Additionally, humans are not able to process large amounts of phenylalanine, and excessive phenylalanine ingestion has been linked to headaches, hypertension and irritability.

Sucralose (aka Splenda)

Sucralose is made from processed sugar. During the food processing the sucrose molecule is replaced by three chlorine atoms. Some studies done with rodents suggest that sucralose may shrink thymus glands, enlarge livers, and cause kidney disorders. THE HEALTH RISKS OF LONG-TERM SUCRALOSE USE IS UNKNOWN. Some former users of sucralose claim that sucralose caused them diarrhea and/or prevented them from losing weight.

Saccharin (aka Sweet 'N Low, Sweet Twin, Necta Sweet)

Saccharin used to carry this warning on its label: "Use of this product may be hazardous to your health. This product contains saccharin which has been determined to cause cancer in laboratory animals." The powerful companies that use or produce this substance have successfully lobbied politicians to stop requiring that they put this warning on the label of products that contain saccharin. I wouldn't use it.

Acesulfame-Potassium (aka Acesulfame-K , Sunette, Sweet One)

This is a relatively new sweetener and there have been relatively few studies done on it. Chemically speaking, acesulfame potassium is the potassium salt of 6-methyl-1,2,3-oxathiazine-4-one 2,2-dioxide. Clearly many more unbiased studies need to be performed on this sweetener before its potential dangers can be assessed. Antidotal reports have already associated acesulfame-potassium with headaches, "cloudy" thinking, nausea, distorted vision, liver problems, kidney problems, and even cancer.

Stevia
Stevia is a South American herb. It has no calories (does not contain sugar) and is believed to be 100 times sweeter than sugar. Stevia may lower hypertension (Chan, 1998 & 2000). Stevia may help lower elevated blood sugar levels. The stevioside in stevia may help to prevent insulin resistance and increase insulin sensitivity (Gregersen, S., et al, 2004). Pure stevia is fine. Be certain, however, to check the ingredients list on any stevia product you wish to purchase to be certain that no other sweeteners have been added. Most readily-available stevia products contain maltodextrin which can elevate blood sugar levels and cause elevated insulin levels. I buy my stevia powder directly from organic farmers who grow the herb (some of these growers sell over the internet). When I find the time I will probably get around to growing my own stevia.

Sugar Alcohol Based Sweeteners (aka Sorbitol, Erythritol, Xylitol, Mannitol)
The main complaint from sugar alcohol users is diarrhea, gas and bloating. While Xylitol derived from birch trees is okay, I wouldn't recommend that anyone suffering with IBS eat any products containing sugar alcohol.

The Threat: Wheat, White Flour and other Grains
Another huge irritant to your intestines are grains. Despite all of the recent propaganda telling us how "healthy" whole grains are for us, the fact is that grains often irritate your body, leading to skin rashes (such as eczema) or intestinal discomfort. Gluten-containing grains can cause Irritable Bowel Syndrome, flatulence and may worsen the symptoms of autism (Whitely, P., et al, 1999). Human beings did not evolve to eat grain. Grain has only been considered a food since the development of agriculture about 10,000 years ago. The nutrients in grains can be found in many other foods. Avoiding grains means avoiding wheat, rye, barley, rice, and corn (which is a grain). These grains are regularly found in bread, pasta, pastry, cakes, biscuits, pies, tarts, breakfast cereals, and anything made out of corn. If you are overweight, and you regularly consume grains, you will almost certainly experience dramatic weight loss by cutting grains out of your diet. I realize that some people with IBS are able to eat a little toast, oatmeal or

crackers without problems, but I just want you to be aware of some of the ways that grains can irritate your intestines and body.

Most processed foods made out of wheat are actually made out of enriched wheat flour, which is a refined product containing several unwholesome ingredients and offering very little nutrition or fiber. When you make flour out of a grain you nearly triple the amount of calories per gram while reducing the amount of beneficial phytonutrients. Enriched wheat flour, rye, and barley contain gluten, and are high in starch, both of which are inflammatory in the body. Many people, such as those with Celiac disease and those of European descent, are gluten-intolerant, and wheat is also a major allergen because it contains the glycoprotein gliadin, which can cause skin rashes such as eczema (my eczema was magically cured when I stopped eating grain and peanuts).

Grains also contain phytic acid which inhibits your body's absorption of important minerals such as iron and magnesium. By soaking, sprouting and/or fermenting grain you can cause the grain to release the enzyme phytase, which will prevent the phytic acid from impeding your body's absorption of minerals (I talk more about this in the next chapter). Unfortunately, most commercial grains have not been properly processed, and may even contain an added enzyme inhibitor which makes them even less healthy for you.

The Threat: "White" foods
For the sake of simplicity I want to use the term "white foods" to help you remember to not eat a lot of the following foods: russet potatoes, salt, refined sugar, white rice, pasta and white flour. Potatoes (especially the ubiquitous Russet Potato) and sugar are full of calories and low in nutrients - the opposite of the kind of nutrient-dense food that we should be eating. The daily average intake of sodium each day by people in America is estimated to be about 3,600 milligrams, but many Americans are eating about three times that amount (microwavable dinners are often loaded with sodium). I would recommend eating between 750 to 2,000 milligrams of unrefined salt a day (I occasionally add Himalayan sea salt to food). We've already talked about the reasons to avoid sugar, white rice, pasta (which is usually derived from grain) and white flour. Try to avoid refined (table) salt altogether and boycott these other bad "white foods" whenever possible.

The Threat: Pasteurized Milk and other Pasteurized Dairy Products

Another food group that can also cause cramping and worsen IBS symptoms is dairy products. If you pay close attention to how you feel after eating pasteurized milk or cheese you will almost certainly feel the negative effects of these foods. Almost all of the milk sold in stores in America has been pasteurized and homogenized. The pasteurization process usually involves heating the milk to a temperature of around 145 degrees Fahrenheit. The beneficial nutrients in milk start becoming denatured and unusable at wet-heat temperatures above 118 degrees Fahrenheit. Additionally, almost all of the beneficial bacteria are destroyed and the naturally occurring enzyme in the milk, lactase, is destroyed. This is why so many people are labeled "lactose intolerant." The sugar in milk is lactose; you need the lactase enzyme to digest lactose. When you eat lactose without having lactase present it can, and usually will, cause cramping and gas. Many people, especially as they grow older, are unable to produce significant amounts of lactase in their bodies and the naturally occurring lactase that was in the milk is destroyed by the pasteurization process. People who are "lactose intolerant" can often drink raw milk without any problems.

Besides being pasteurized almost all of the milk sold in stores is homogenized as well. The homogenization process essentially forces the milk through such tiny holes at such high pressure that the milk will not separate again (the cream will not float on top of the milk). Some people interested in health believe that homogenization is even worse than pasteurization, in part because it allows the xanthine oxidase content of cow milk to be absorbed into the body. During the homogenization process the butterfat is changed into spheres of fat containing xanthine oxidase, and this powerful enzyme can create wounds throughout your body as it circulates through your blood stream.

Similarly, I don't consider any cheese that is made out of pasteurized milk to be a particularly healthy food, especially for people suffering from any kind of bowel discomfort. Commercial yogurts usually consist of sugar, some genetically modified corn extracts (starch or high fructose corn syrup), and some type of preservative mixed into a base of pasteurized dairy. Some even contain artificial colors and/or flavors. Commercial yogurts are not particularly good for you. They contain such a small amount of beneficial bacteria (probiotics) that you would have to eat about 30 servings to equal the bacteria count of one quality probiotic capsule.

Humans have been using various substances to help preserve their foods for a long time, but in the past people used natural preservatives. Nowadays food manufacturers are routinely using chemical preservatives that have been shown to have negative effects on one's health. The health hazards of chemical preservatives range from causing headaches to causing cancer (Rogers, M. A., et al, 1995).

Some of the more common preservatives to watch out for, and avoid, include: Thiabendazole, sodium benzoate, benzoic acid, sorbic acid, bromates (commonly found in white flour and bread), brominated oils, mono-glycerides and di-glycerides, propyl gallate, sulfites, parabens, maleic hydrazide, propylene glycol (also used to make antifreeze), carboxymethylcellulose, sulfur dioxide, biphenyl (aka diphenyl), and sodium nitrate.

Sodium nitrate is often used to preserve ham, bacon, hot dogs, sausage, bologna, "deli" meat, "sandwich" meat, and other processed meats. Sodium nitrate is often converted into nitrosamine by your body, and nitrosamine is a serious carcinogen. Sodium nitrate is so dangerous that both Germany and Norway have listed nitrates as outright toxins and completely banned them. Foods like beer and cheese usually contain nitrosamine.

Another thing to be aware of is that pharmaceutical antibiotics kill the good bacteria in your body (the probiotics), leaving an environment that can easily become a breeding ground for bad bacteria and candida yeast overgrowth. These conditions alone can cause irritable bowel syndrome. The colon-cleansing protocols discussed in this book, together with eating significant amounts of probiotics on a regular basis, can help to repopulate your good bacteria and kill or remove bad bacteria. If candida yeast has overpopulated your intestines, however, you may have to go on a sugar-free diet and take supplements that fight yeast. Some yeast-fighting supplements include caprylic acid, garlic, pau d'arco and enzymes like cellulase that digest yeast cell walls. I had a bad case of candida yeast overgrowth, but I got rid of the problem and I feel a LOT better now!

How to Feel Great, Stay Healthy, and Have Energy

I can summarize an entire healthy regimen in one sentence: Eat organic, whole foods, as raw as possible, and only when you're actually hungry. I'm sure that you've heard *someone* talking about "juicing" at some point during your life. There are reasons why you heard that and why juicing isn't going away any time soon. When people who have been eating the Standard American Diet of processed, chemical-laden foods start eating whole, nutrient-dense, relatively toxin-free organic food their energy and mental focus can improve dramatically. That's why you occasionally hear someone raving about juicing. In her book "Green for Life," Victoria Boutenko describes what happened when she got about forty people together and asked them to replace one meal a day with a green smoothie. A green smoothie is just fruit and greens (like lettuce, spinach, kale, parsley, celery...etc.) put in a blender or juicer. Each participant that stayed on the plan had more energy, increased sex drive, slept better, lowered their cholesterol, reduced body inflammation and lost weight. You don't even need to buy a juicer to "juice" most vegetables. I've been using a good, high speed blender to mix up my lettuce, spinach, kale, parsley, beet leaves, chard, apples, bananas, berries and ginger for years now.

Not to worry, you don't *have* to start juicing or blending up things. I do, however, highly recommend that you start to eat "cleaner," and that does require you to eat more of the foods that nature intended you to eat. There's a price to pay for eating foods that are not in their natural state (processed foods), and that price is usually disease. So before, during and after the time you are cleaning your colon, you should eat some good fresh organic fruit and vegetables. A high colonic cleans your large intestine quite thoroughly, but the best way to get and keep your entire digestive tract clean from the top down, is to eat healthy foods.

IBS sufferers should eat some soluble fiber before eating a meal. I remember when I had IBS I used to wake up in the morning and take some psyllium husk powder. It did help me start my day cramp-free, but psyllium husk doesn't agree with everyone's system. Other foods that contain soluble fiber include oatmeal, apples and bananas, so you might want to start your day with one of those foods.

Fruit actually helps keep your colon healthy by providing fiber, pectin, antioxidants and other nutrients. Fruit is easy to digest and should be eaten alone so that your body can move it through your colon quickly without any competing starches or proteins. One of the most important things to know about eating healthy is to know when to eat what. Some foods don't mix well at all. For example, starches (like potatoes and rice) shouldn't be eaten with protein because the starches digest well in a stomach that's not too acidic, but proteins need a lot of that hydrochloric acid (HCL) acidity in order for the amino acids in them to be fully digested. Proteins also don't digest well with fats. I usually try to eat proteins only with non or low starch vegetables like various greens, and I always eat fruit alone.

One of the easiest ways to not mix incompatible food types is to divide up your meals throughout the day.   When you eat a lot of food all at once there is also a larger spike in your blood sugar level, which doesn't benefit most people. I suggest eating about five or six smaller meals a day, and again, only eat when you are actually hungry, don't eat according to a clock. I have gotten to the point where I can tell whether my body wants a carbohydrate meal or a protein meal just by the way the hunger feels. Ask your body if it would rather eat a steak OR a potato and listen to its answer. Hey, steak AND potatoes wasn't one of the options!

Here is a list of healthy, IBS-friendly foods...

EVERYTHING IS CERTIFIED ORGANIC WHENEVER POSSIBLE - NO PESTICIDES OR GENETICALLY MODIFIED ORGANISMS (GMO's) !

Recommended Proteins:

Legumes
Kidney beans
Chicken, turkey, duck or quail (baked & skinless)
Egg whites
Fish - only if it is a very low mercury variety of fish caught in the arctic or other relatively pristine part of the world
Cheese (raw only unless taking lactase enzyme)
Cottage cheese
Beef (grass-fed only)
Bison

Rabbit
Lamb

Recommended Fats:

Avocados
Coconuts, coconut oil and raw coconut butter
Eggs (eat the yolk only if it doesn't cause you gas)
Nuts (raw only)
Fish - only if it is very low in mercury
Olives and extra-virgin olive oil
Cod liver oil
Seeds (raw)
Flax seeds
Chia seeds

Recommended vegetables:

Asparagus
Bean sprouts
Celery
Chicory leaves
Chives
Cucumber
Endive
Fennel bulb
Green Beans
Gourd (calabash)
Kale
Lettuce
Mung beans (sprouted)
Mushrooms (okay, it's actually a mold)
Mustard greens
Okra
Onions
Peas

Peppers (sweet)
Radishes
Rhubarb
Sauerkraut (ease into it)
Spinach
Spirulina (really an alga)
Spring greens
Squash (summer)
Swiss chard
Tomato (fresh)
Turnip greens
Zucchini

Recommended Fruit:

Note: Pay close attention to how your gut feels after eating fruit. Do you experience bloating, or abdominal cramps or pain? Some people do not digest fructose (fruit sugar) well, and then the fruit essentially ferments, causing gas-producing bacteria. If you experience these symptoms it's best to limit the amount of sugar, including fructose, in your diet. Remember that you should eat fruit all by itself and not mix it with other foods.

Apples
Apricots
Avocados
Bananas
most berries (i.e. blueberries, raspberries, goji berries, acai berries...etc.)
Mangoes
Noni
Oranges, lemons and most citrus
Papayas
Raisins

Make sure that you get plenty of soluble and insoluble fiber. Fiber helps fecal matter move through your intestines. If you're eating a lot of whole fruit and vegetables you will get a good amount of fiber in your diet.

I understand that the above list of foods may not look anything like what you are actually eating, but I'm honestly just trying to tell you what will help you the most. I admit that I eat quite a bit of rice in order to help me avoid wheat (like rice bagels). You should make a slow, deliberate transition into a healthy, whole foods diet. Identify the worst foods you currently eat and decide to eliminate them, one per week, until you have replaced the vast majority of your unhealthy choices with healthy alternatives. If you switch from a typical American food diet to a healthy diet all at once you will suffer from detoxification symptoms. When you start giving your body more energy it will use some of that energy to purge toxins. This results in an increase in the amount of toxins moving through your blood for a while. Overall this is a good thing as the toxins are ultimately on their way out of your body, but you should ease into this detoxification by not doing too much all at once. Whenever I detoxify my body I take supplements to support my liver because that is your body's main filter. These liver-friendly supplements include milk thistle, methylsulfonylmethane (MSM), and N-acetyl-L-cysteine (NAC).

You should drink about half a gallon of water a day. Water makes up nearly 85 percent of your brain and about 80 percent of your blood. I avoid tap water because it often contains some of the following toxins: chlorine, fluoride, chromium-6, perchlorates, benzene, MTBE, trichloroethylene, trihalomethanes, radon, arsenic, lead and a host of other heavy metals and chemicals. Bottled water is usually packaged in plastic that can contain Bis-phenol A (BPA), Bis-phenol B (BPB), PVC, estrogenic chemicals, and antimony (a toxic chemical element that can cause headaches, dizziness and depression). According to some estimates Americans throw away about 95,000,000 plastic bottles every day. I drink filtered (like reverse osmosis), remineralized (I add beneficial minerals such as magnesium and fulvic minerals back into the water that is now virtually devoid of all minerals) water throughout the day. Dehydration can cause constipation, and it is estimated that about 75% of Americans are chronically dehydrated. It's best to drink water in-between meals as opposed to drinking a lot of liquid while eating. Soda, alcohol, energy drinks, caffeinated beverages and commercial fruit juices should be minimized or avoided altogether.

Many people I know personally seem to be thriving on a predominantly (NOT completely) raw-food diet. The main benefit of a raw food diet is that, not only are all of the nutrients present and non-denatured, but the naturally-occurring enzymes in the food are still usable by your body. This is a huge thing. As previously mentioned, your body requires digestive enzymes to digest food, and if the food you eat doesn't contain the enzymes in a usable form, your pancreas has to work to manufacture it (if it can!). This takes energy from your body. If I plan to eat a meal consisting of cooked food I will usually take a digestive enzyme capsule before eating. Another benefit of eating raw foods is that the glutathione in the food has not been destroyed by cooking. Glutathione is arguably the most important antioxidant in your body. Other antioxidants such as vitamins C and E cannot even work if glutathione is not present. In addition to helping our immune systems stay strong, glutathione helps protect the mitochondria of our cells which power our entire bodies. Perhaps you've heard that the energy in food comes from the sun. This is due to the fact that plants derive their energy from the sun, and animals eat plants (or animals eat animals that eat plants). When you are eating uncooked plants you are much closer to the original energy source of the sun. From my viewpoint, the longer you cook foods or the higher up on the food chain the food is, the less "life" energy there is left in the food. A healthy raw diet consists of a lot of uncooked plant food, such as vegetables, fruits, nuts and seeds. Eating raw is not expensive and actually saves you time by eliminating the need for cooking. A raw diet tends to increase your energy because the foods are easy to digest and may contain more life force. Most raw food diets will help resolve digestive issues, reduce food allergies (just pay close attention to how you're reacting to nuts), strengthen your immune system, and lower your cholesterol if it truly is too high. Many people who include more raw foods in their diet report developing more attractive, radiant skin, stronger hair and nails and experiencing less depression or fatigue. If you are overweight a raw diet will help you quickly move towards your ideal weight. If an overweight person ate a raw meal each day instead of eating a typical American meal he or she would probably lose pounds of weight each week. The fiber in fruits and vegetables help you feel full, and the nutrients in them satisfy your body's needs so it doesn't continue to crave more food. Many raw foodists rely on their juicers or blenders to liquefy items such as spinach, lettuce, celery, parsley, kale, apples, and ginger so they can drink their meals easily. It's actually good to break up the food you eat into little pieces because it creates more surface area for your digestive enzymes to work on - food processors essentially pre-chew the food for you. Just don't over-blend delicate greens because you will oxidize the chlorophyll in them. I regularly go out into my garden first thing in the morning, harvest some "greens" like lettuce, kale, chard and/or purslane, and juice them up into an incredibly energizing breakfast; I add in whey protein from grass-fed cows, and coconut butter and non-GMO lecithin, among other things.

Raw nuts are one of the staples of a raw food diet. I don't recommend some nuts, such as peanuts, because they're too high in omega-6 (and are subject to being contaminated with aflatoxin from the Aspergillus flavus fungus). But even raw nuts should be soaked before eating because nuts are seeds, and their hulls contain enzyme inhibitors that inhibit digestion. You want enzyme activity in your stomach because that's how your body begins breaking down and absorbing nutrients from the food you eat. So to significantly reduce the amount of naturally occurring enzyme inhibitors on nuts you should soak them in water (with a little sea salt in it) for a few hours before eating them or actually sprout them. Pecans, almonds and walnuts should soak for about 12 hours (I usually just let them soak overnight), flax seeds, sesame seeds, pumpkin seeds and hazel nuts should soak about 8 hours, cashews, brazil nuts, sunflower seeds, pistachios, and macadamias should soak for 4 hours and pine nuts and chia seeds should be soaked for about 2 hours. After soaking the nuts, rinse the nuts to wash any remaining water they were sitting in off of the nuts. Some people dry soaked nuts in an oven set to 150 degrees or use a dehydrator to dry them. I usually just eat them wet.

Grains also contain an enzyme inhibitor called phytic acid. If you soak your whole grains in water overnight you will encourage the grain to produce phytase which helps neutralizes the phytic acid. To further reduce phytic acid one should actually sprout the grain and ferment it. Since these processes are almost never done with commercial grains it is best to avoid most commercial grains. It's a lot of work to soak grain, dry it, ground it, ferment it using water or an acidic medium (such as unpasteurized apple cider vinegar, yogurt, or kefir) and let it set for 36 hours before baking it.

Although it's not always convenient to find or create fermented foods they are critically important to maintaining good health because they help maintain a healthy gut flora. Gut flora (or microflora) refers to the trillions of microorganisms that live in our digestive tracts. It is estimated that about 500 different species of bacteria live in a typical adult human. The goal is to have a colon that is full of helpful microorganisms while keeping your pathogenic bacteria count down.

Maintaining Your Cure

Using the advice in this book I am confident that you will be able to get your IBS under control in a single season. During the process of healing, however, your IBS attack symptoms may very well try to return occasionally. Don't keep your eye on the calendar; keep your focus on the cures. The object isn't to forget you ever had IBS; the object is to accept that part of your life as natural and okay. Good health is based on a good relationship between you and your body. Keep yourself emotionally balanced. Get into the habit of monitoring the level of stress in your body and catch yourself if you're running any bad thoughts in your mind. Attitude is important. Stress can interfere with your ability to have a healthy colon, and an unhealthy colon can cause you to have stress. Remember that the majority of your serotonin is produced in your gut, so a healthy gut helps to reduce stress. If you are suffering from a great deal of emotional stress in your life you will have more difficulty healing your intestines, so take the time to identify the stressors in your life and employ actions to remove or reduce their impact.

One good habit to get into is to schedule some quiet time for yourself each day. There are many things that you can use to help you reduce stress, improve yourself and help you maintain a positive outlook. Here is a list of some of those things:

MEDITATION is a wonderful tool. Some people use it to promote spiritual growth or find inner peace, while others use it as a relaxation and stress-reduction tool. Don't think that you need to study how to meditate. All you have to do is find a nice, quiet place free from distractions. You can sit on the floor cross-legged, lie down on a bed, couch or floor or get in whatever other position feels comfortable. Just take nice, deep breaths in and slowly let your breath out. Focus on your breathing. Pay no mind to any other thoughts your mind has. Keep returning your mental focus to your breath and the inside of your body. You can visualize a white or gold light flowing into or through your body with every breath. Some people visualize the light flowing in through the top of their head (crown point) and some people visualize the light as something they breathe in through their mouth. Some people imagine the light flowing out through their feet (bubbling spring point) and some people visualize a dark cloud of bad thoughts, emotions or energy exiting their bodies through their mouth as they breathe out. Visualize your intestines healing. Just be there for about 15 minutes a day with yourself and see what you start feeling. Go with that feeling. If you identify any deep, underlying emotional problems or personality flaws you can use tools like meditation to help heal the root cause. You can listen to guided meditations that will tell you what to do step by step.

BACH FLOWER ESSENCES consist of a homeopathic dilution of flower essences in water and alcohol. There is no significant amount of any drug or chemical in them besides the alcohol. I used to think that homeopathic medicines were a hoax before I actually took some and was miraculously cured of some ailments. Some books on quantum physics state that all objects, including people, are composed of slightly over 99.9 percent empty space. This is because atoms consist of 99.9+% empty space and we are made out of atoms. An atom has a nucleus and electrons, but in the space between them there is no detectable matter, only energy. We are comprised mostly of energy, making us beings of energy. Homeopathic medicine works on an energy level. If you are able to identify some chronic emotions in yourself like anger, worry, impatience, or fearfulness you can use the appropriate Bach flower remedy to help avoid experiencing that emotion. I have used several of these essences and have found them to be very helpful.

HAVING A PURPOSE-DRIVEN LIFE makes you eager to get out of bed in the morning. Find a life purpose that inspires you. Get involved. What is important to you? What are you passionate about? We're waiting!

EMOTIONAL FREEING TECHNIQUE (EFT) is a form of psychological acupuncture that uses light tapping with your fingertips, instead of inserting needles, to stimulate traditional Chinese acupuncture points. The tapping on these designated points on the head and body is combined with verbalizing the identified problem, followed by a general affirmation phrase. This technique is designed to relieve stress, abolish phobias, stop food cravings and reduce pain and discomfort. I have used this technique with positive results. Look for a book called "2 Minute EFT Meridian Tapping Routines for Wealth Health Love Happiness and Everything Else!"

T'AI CHI & CHI GUNG (QIGONG). T'ai Chi is a form of Chi Gung. Although T'ai Chi is better known in America, I actually practice Chi Gung more often. Chi Gung improves physical functioning, alleviates symptoms of depression and anxiety, and lowers blood pressure in adults. It is not strenuous and can be done by people of all ages. Chi Gung has been proven to improve the physical health of middle-aged women. It also works on men as well. I have felt the amazing power of Chi Gung and it has changed my life. With practice you can feel the chi (life energy) in your body and significantly increase this, and your, energy!

THERAPISTS can listen to you and help you work through your emotional issues. I recommend that you seek out a talented naturopath, homeopath or psychologist. Although psychologists can prescribe drugs in some states, they do not usually rely on them to "treat" their patients like psychiatrists do. A person could be a good counselor to you even if they don't have a college degree on the wall.

PHYSICAL EXERCISE helps keep both your mind and body healthy. A workout could be playing tennis, golfing, cooking, exercising to a video, walking, gardening, dynamic stretching or whatever you like to do to move your body. Moderate exercise is a great way to reduce the amount of stress in your body and get rid of "nervous energy."

DEEP BREATHING brings oxygen into your body and helps you expel stress. Your emotional and mental states are closely linked to your breathing patterns. When people start feeling anxious their breath usually starts getting shallower. Most people breathe too shallow throughout their lives. You can teach yourself to get in the habit of breathing deeply by practicing deep breathing exercises (Chi Gung is wonderful for this). Controlling your breath controls your mental state, allowing you to manage your stress, panic and anxiety. Breathe deeply from your abdomen, observing how your muscles contract and expand as you breathe. Slowly inhale through your nose and focus on filling your lungs from the bottom to the very top. Hold your breath for a few seconds before slowly breathing out through your mouth while visualizing the air coming from the top of the lungs and slowly flattening your lungs out to their bottoms.

GET IN NATURE and reconnect. Take a walk. Get some glorious sun. Pet a cat or dog. Nature is waiting to heal you.

YOGA is like moving meditation. Yoga can relax your body and put your mind into measurably different brain wave patterns. It's a wonderful way to relieve stress and anxiety and promote overall health.

NURTURING CLOSE, PERSONAL RELATIONSHIPS has been consistently shown to increase satisfaction with one's life. Be available when your friends need you. Be a good listener and offer others what you can. With today's technology it's easy to stay in touch with people through the phone or e-mail. A study was conducted at Brigham Young University that concluded that "having a larger social network of friends, family, and colleagues can increase your chances of being alive by as much as 50 percent!" (Holt-Lunstad, Smith).

FENG SHU is an ancient method that helps ensure that the life force, Qi (pronounced "chee" in English), flows through your environment. The orientation of a building, its age, and its interaction with the surrounding environment, including which way doors face, affects the flow of Qi. I know this sounds like nonsense to some people but I would simply say "Try it!" If you ever feel like the energy just gets taken out of you when you enter a certain room in your house that room would be the place to start. Make space and open the room up. Move things away from doorways so energy can better enter into the room. Move furniture against the wall and keep the center of the room clutter-free. If you do it right, you will *feel* the difference in your energy and it will improve the happiness level of your mind. Try it!

Other therapies include getting negative ions from the air, relaxation exercises, acupuncture, acupressure, listening to relaxing music, massage, and napping.

I sincerely hope that I have been of significant service to you and helped you on your way to end any and all of your abdominal discomfort. Have faith, not just in yourself, but in the world. You don't have to figure everything out yourself. You don't have to do everything yourself. The Universe, your own body, nature and other caring people are waiting to help and to heal you. Listen to your heart, live in gratitude, look for the humor in things, decide to be happy, and make your life wonderful

This book is for informational purposes only. The statements made in this book have not been evaluated by the FDA and are not intended to diagnose, treat, cure or prevent any disease. Anyone suffering with any medical condition should see a qualified medical professional to correctly identify the causes. Neither the author nor The Natural Cure Network has received any incentive, monetary or otherwise, to endorse or mention any specific product companies. No part of this book can be reproduced or distributed without the written permission of the Natural Cure Network. © Copyright 2012, 2013 Natural Cure Network, Inc.

www.ingramcontent.com/pod-product-compliance
Lightning Source LLC
Chambersburg PA
CBHW071343310526
45790CB00018B/1201

* 9 7 8 1 4 8 4 0 3 3 5 0 0 *